KNOWING ABOUT DIABETES

For Insulin-Dependent Diabetics

Dr. P. H. Wise MB PhD, FRCP FRACP

Consultant Physician
Diabetic and Endocrine Clinic
Charing Cross Hospital, London

Second Edition

foulsham
LONDON • NEW YORK • TORONTO • SYDNEY

foulsham
Yeovil Road, Slough, Berkshire, SL1 4JH

ISBN 0–572–02020–1
Copyright © 1983 & 1994 P. H. Wise

In this book, the author and editor have done their best to outline the
indicated general treatment for Diabetes (Insulin Dependent).
Recommendations are made regarding certain drugs, medications and
preparations.

Different people react to the same treatment, medication, or
preparation in different ways. This book does not purport to answer all
questions about all situations that you or your child may encounter. It
does not attempt to replace your physician.

Neither the editors nor the publishers of this book take responsibility
for any possible consequences from any treatment, action or application
of any medication or preparation to any person reading or following the
information or advice contained in this book. The publication of this
book does not constitute the practice of medicine. The author and
publisher advise that you consult your physician before administering
any medication or undertaking any course of treatment.

Printed in Great Britain by
St Edmundsbury Press Ltd, Bury St Edmunds, Suffolk

INTRODUCTION:

You may have had diabetes for some time: perhaps you already know much of what is in this book. On the other hand, the diagnosis may have just been made, and all that is involved may seem a little bewildering.

This book was written to give you some idea of what diabetes is all about. It tries to answer the type of questions you will ask, both now and in the future. It cannot cover the whole subject, and at the end you will find a list of books for further reading.

There is one thing that most authorities agree upon: the more that diabetics know, the better controlled and the healthier they are likely to be. Never hesitate to ask for additional information and help.

ACKNOWLEDGEMENTS:

The author acknowledges with appreciation the constructive criticism of the many patients, nurses and other health professionals who helped to produce this book. Special thanks go to Eleanor McGill who provided nutritional information for this book.

1 WHAT IS DIABETES?

Diabetes is the name given to a disturbed chemical balance in the body, which can affect a number of different organs. The word diabetes comes from a Greek expression meaning "siphon". It refers to the increased urination and thirst which often occurs in newly diagnosed or uncontrolled cases. These symptoms are due to the high sugar (glucose) content in the urine. This in turn results from an excessive build-up of glucose in the blood.

Diabetes is due to partial or complete lack of insulin. This hormone is normally released directly into the blood circulation from small pockets of cells called Islets of Langerhans, which are scattered throughout the pancreas gland (sweetbread). The pancreas rests in the upper abdomen, just beneath the liver, partly behind the stomach in the loop of the duodenum.

The pancreas also produces enzymes, which pass through a duct into the duodenum, where

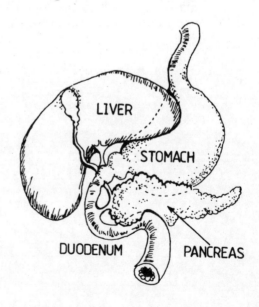

LIVER

STOMACH

DUODENUM   PANCREAS

they assist with the digestion of food. This part of the pancreas is only rarely affected in diabetes.

Insulin in usable form was first extracted from animal pancreas in 1921 by two Canadians, Banting and Best. Shortly afterwards it proved successful in the treatment of human diabetes.

About one person in every fifty is diabetic, although only one in four diabetics actually needs insulin for treatment.

2/ WHAT DOES INSULIN NORMALLY DO?

Insulin has many different effects, helping the body to manufacture proteins, fats and other substances. However, its main action is to encourage glucose in the blood to enter the cells of all major body tissues. In these tissues, it can be stored (as a substance called glycogen in liver and muscle cells). It can also be used as fuel to create energy. This energy can be used to speed up almost every chemical process in the body. If insufficient insulin is produced, the body accordingly malfunctions in a number of ways. Furthermore, since the glucose is not being used by the cells, it builds up in the blood to a level which is above normal. This is called **hyperglycaemia**.

3/ HOW DOES UNCONTROLLED DIABETES (HYPERGLYCAEMIA) PRODUCE SYMPTOMS?

When blood glucose rises above normal (see Question 21), a number of things may happen:

a) In the early stages, or if the rise of blood glucose is only moderate, **there may be no**

symptoms at all. As the glucose level rises higher, one or more of the following may occur:

b) The lens of the eye may alter its shape, producing **blurring of vision**.

c) High glucose levels in the blood reduce the body's defences against infection. Skin, urine, lung and other **infections** may therefore occur. In fact, it may be just such an infection which first alerted your doctor that you might have diabetes.

d) More glucose in the blood can interfere with brain activity, affecting **concentration** and causing **lethargy**.

e) By overflowing into the urine (where it is usually first tested), glucose may draw water with it: **more urine** is then passed.

f) Excessive urination reduces the body's fluid reserves and stimulates **thirst** in an attempt to keep body fluid supplies normal.

g) The passing of excessive urine also results in loss of essential chemicals (sodium, potassium and magnesium), producing **cramps, tiredness** and **weakness**.

h) Because glucose cannot be properly used by the body and is lost in the urine, the body uses its stores of fat as a fuel supply, resulting in **weight loss**.

i) If very severe loss of fluid occurs, the body becomes dry (**dehydrated**): **breathlessness** and even **coma** may then occur.

j) Prolonged high levels of blood glucose, even if taking insulin, can damage body tissues over a period of years. This can lead to the so-called **complications** of diabetes (see Questions 29 and 30).

WHY DOES DIABETES DEVELOP?
There are different types of diabetes, but in most patients the the tendency to diabetes is partly inherited from one or both sides of the family. However, there are almost always additional factors which are responsible for setting the disorder in motion.

In the more late-developing (non-insulin-dependent or maturity-onset) diabetes, insulin deficiency is only mild. In such cases diabetes may show up because of being overweight, or may result from the effects of repeated pregnancy, certain drugs, stress or just ageing itself.

However, **in your type of diabetes**, whatever your age, the lack of insulin has become more severe or even total, perhaps resulting from additional severe damage to the pancreas gland by a virus, or from other factors which we cannot yet identify. Therefore your diabetes is referred to as either insulin-requiring or insulin-dependent diabetes. Accordingly, only insulin itself can be used for treatment.

 DOES DIABETES EVER GO AWAY?
No. It can always be controlled and with treatment you should feel completely well. Even when treated, however, it must still be carefully watched by you and regularly reviewed by your doctor for the rest of your life.

6 WHAT ARE THE MAJOR AIMS AND PRINCIPLES OF DIABETIC TREATMENT?

The first aim of treating your diabetes is to keep your blood glucose level as close as is practical to that of a non-diabetic person. By this and other means, the second aim can be achieved: to minimise or avoid the so-called complications of diabetes. There is a lot of research both from Europe and the USA which clearly shows that the more normal you keep your blood sugar, the less likely it is that you will develop these longer-term complications.

There are three essential principles for achieving good control: **diet, insulin and exercise**. The diet needs to provide a nutritious source of energy which is reasonably constant from day to day. The food you eat also needs to be accurately matched to a dose of insulin, which is usually injected twice or more daily.

Exercise helps to keep body weight constant but in addition lowers the blood glucose level in a very similar way to insulin.

7 HOW IS FOOD NORMALLY PROCESSED BY THE BODY AND WHAT GOES WRONG IN DIABETES?

Foods, which are all different mixtures of carbohydrates, proteins, and fats, provide the body with energy. The energy value of any diet is expressed as calories:

One gram of carbohydrate provides four calories

One gram of protein provides four calories

One gram of fat provides nine calories

One gram of pure alcohol provides seven calories

Food also contains essential minerals and vitamins, but these do not provide the body with usable energy. Depending on age, weight and physical activity, the energy needs of the body range between 1000 and 4000 calories per day.

After eating a meal, food passes into the stomach where it is digested (broken down) into smaller particles. Partly digested food then passes into the small intestine where digestion is completed and the small particles pass through the wall of the intestine into the blood stream.

The digested nutrients (carbohydrate, protein and fat) are carried to the liver where they may all be converted into glucose under some circumstances: however, most glucose comes direct from carbohydrate. Consequently, after a meal (especially if it is high in carbohydrate), there is a rise in the amount of glucose in the blood. The following diagram will give you an idea of the normal variation of blood glucose in a non-diabetic person.

In non-diabetics, a rise of blood glucose stimulates the pancreas to produce and release more insulin into the blood vessels which pass through the pancreas. From here, the insulin is distributed to the liver and all other body

Normal variation of blood glucose in a non-diabetic person.

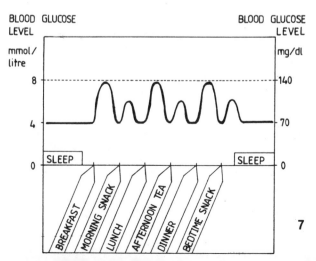

7

tissues. In this way, the glucose level is lowered back to normal within two hours, by forcing glucose to pass into body cells where it is processed to produce energy. If energy is not needed immediately, insulin allows glucose to be stored in muscles or liver in the form of another carbohydrate called glycogen (to be used when extra energy is needed), or promotes the production of fat (for more long-term storage). Insulin also stimulates the formation of proteins, important for the development of muscle, bone, and other supporting tissues.

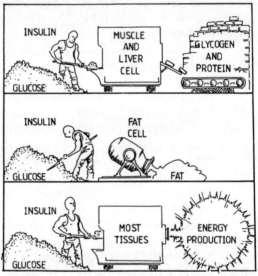

Different tissues use glucose for different purposes

Because diabetics do not produce sufficient insulin, the blood glucose level is high even if no food is eaten. This is because the body makes glucose from its own carbohydrates, proteins, and fats. After a meal the blood glucose level goes even higher, and the glucose is partly removed from the blood by escaping through the kidneys into the urine. Furthermore, since the body cannot use the glucose properly to produce energy, such energy must be obtained by other means: from the breakdown of fat stores and protein-rich tissues in the body. This process leads to the loss of weight and ill health of uncontrolled diabetes.

WHAT ARE THE PRINCIPLES OF DIABETIC DIETS?

A diabetic diet is a healthy, balanced diet: the sort of diet that is recommended for everyone (although very young children and babies have special requirements). Why not convert your family and friends? Discussion with your dietitian, perhaps also involving some members of your family will inform you of foods which are particular to your likes and needs, whatever your ethnic or national background. However, there are six basic principles which all people with diabetes should follow to keep their diabetes well controlled.

a) Avoid sugar and sugary foods

We are talking about sugar, glucose, jam, honey, sweets, chocolates, fizzy drinks, and fruit squashes. The sugar in these foods enters the blood very quickly, causing a rapid rise in blood sugar which is difficult for insulin to deal with. Many foods contain sugar. However, it is only necessary to avoid foods in which sugar is a major ingredient. Check the ingredient label of a food if you are not sure whether it is suitable. The ingredients are listed in order of weight: i.e. sugar at the top of the list means it contains a large amount. If sugar is towards the end of the list, the food is suitable i.e. it contains very little.

b) Eat regularly

You should aim for three meals a day. One or two large meals raise the blood glucose too high and are difficult for insulin to deal with properly. A meal may be as little as a sandwich, or as much as a cooked meal of meat, potatoes and vegetables, followed by dessert. Eating regularly is particularly important to **avoid hypoglycaemia** (low blood sugar). As you can see in Question 11, different insulins have different times of peak action and duration.

The type and dose of insulins you have been prescribed were chosen to suit your lifestyle and requirements. Check with your diabetes nurse, doctor, or dietitian, whether your insulin regimen means that you also need a snack between your meals. Eating a larger meal than usual is fine, on occasions, but you will need to increase your insulin dose before that meal, to prevent the blood glucose from rising too high. Your diabetes nurse, doctor, or dietitian will be able to advise you on this.

c) Eat some starchy food with each meal

We are talking about bread, potatoes, rice, pasta, and breakfast cereal. In earlier years, diabetics were advised to avoid or restrict these foods. We now believe that a good intake of them is important. These foods are broken down into sugar by the body. They are broken down more slowly than sugary foods, causing a slower, smaller rise in blood sugar. These sorts of changes in blood sugar occur in non-diabetic people and are therefore, to some extent, normal. Eat the amount of starchy foods you normally have with a meal: i.e. two slices of bread, two potatoes, etc. A low blood glucose level (see Question 24) may occur if you forget to include these foods in your meals, or try to drastically reduce them. By the same token, if you eat considerably more of them than you normally do, your blood sugar will be higher than usual.

d) Eat less fat and fatty foods

We are including here butter, oil, margarine, fried foods, and pastry of all types. Having a high fat intake increases your risk of suffering from heart attacks or strokes, which are in any case rather more likely to occur in someone with diabetes. Smoking or being overweight increases the risk still further. It makes sense to avoid risks! Cutting down on fat has the added advantage that it automatically reduces your calorie intake, as high fat foods are more fattening than lower fat alternatives. Avoiding high fat foods will therefore help you to reduce your weight, if necessary, or help to prevent you from becoming overweight.

e) **Drink alcohol in moderation**

The safe weekly limits are considered to be 15 drinks (or units) for a woman, or 22 drinks (or units) for a man, spread over the week. One unit is a single pub measure of spirit, an average glass of wine, or a half pint of beer, lager or cider. Alcohol is high in calories and will make you gain weight. It is also bad for your general health (liver, heart, brain, and nerves, in particular) if taken in excess. Too much alcohol at once, especially on an empty stomach, may cause your blood sugar to go too low. **Do not drink alcohol on an empty stomach**, avoid having more than three or four drinks in a session, and follow alcohol with a snack containing at least some starchy food: i.e. a sandwich.

f) **Eat more fibre**

Dietary fibre is the part of a plant which is not digested properly by the body. High fibre foods include wholemeal bread, brown rice, wholegrain pasta, vegetables (especially beans, peas, and lentils) and wholegrain breakfast cereals. Eating high fibre foods with your meals reduces the rise in blood sugar which occurs after eating. High fibre foods can also be helpful in reducing blood fats, i.e. cholesterol, and tend to be very filling. They can therefore be helpful in reducing weight and preventing weight gain. They also help to produce regular bowel movements. Not being overweight has been mentioned many times in this Section. Turn to Question 9 to see the desirable weight for you. It is *very* important that you try to reduce your weight if you are overweight. Diabetes is more difficult to control when you are overweight. If you are having difficulty in losing weight, ask your doctor to refer you to the dietitian. She will draw up an eating plan tailored to your needs which will help you to achieve your weight target.

It is very important to see a dietitian regularly: you will be given a lot of information and no one would expect you to remember it all at your first visit. Furthermore, the diet may need to be changed over a period of time -particularly if you change your way of life, gain weight, or if the type of insulin you use is changed. Check with Question 37 to be sure you have a contact number for your dietitian.

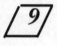

IS WEIGHT CONTROL IMPORTANT?

Yes. Being overweight increases your need for insulin and can make your diabetes less stable. It may also cause or aggravate conditions unrelated to diabetes, such as high blood pressure and arthritis.

The only way you can influence your weight is by diet and exercise (see Question 14). Remember that one extra hour of brisk walking (or half-an-hour of continuous swimming, jogging or squash) each day will almost predictably allow you to lose about 7 kg (15 pounds) in a year - providing you do not increase your food intake! Use the table opposite as a guide to your goal weight.

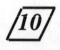

HOW IS INSULIN GIVEN?

Insulin needs to be injected because if taken by mouth the digestive enzymes of the stomach and intestine destroy it before it can be absorbed.

The amount of insulin used in treatment is expressed in units. Insulin is manufactured in various strengths (concentrations) throughout the world, but these days 100 units per ml is the one most often used.

It is important to check your insulin each time it is prescribed and dispensed, to make sure that you have the correct type. It

ADULT DESIRABLE WEIGHT

A weight 2–2.5 kg (5 pounds) above or below is acceptable.

| HEIGHT (without shoes) | | WEIGHT (without clothes) | | | |
| | | MEN | | WOMEN | |
Feet/ Inches	Centi- metres	Pounds	Kilo- grams	Pounds	Kilo- grams
4/10	147.5	—	—	107	48.5
4/11	150.0	—	—	110	50.0
5/0	152.5	—	—	113	51.5
5/1	155.0	—	—	116	52.5
5/2	157.5	129	58.5	119	54.0
5/3	160.0	133	60.5	122	55.5
5/4	162.5	136	62.0	126	57.0
5/5	165.0	139	63.0	130	59.0
5/6	167.5	143	65.0	135	61.0
5/7	170.0	147	66.5	139	63.0
5/8	172.5	152	69.0	143	65.0
5/9	175.5	156	71.0	147	66.5
5/10	178.0	160	72.5	151	68.5
5/11	180.5	165	75.0	155	70.5
6/0	183.0	170	77.0	—	—
6/1	185.5	175	79.5	—	—
6/2	188.0	180	81.5	—	—
6/3	190.5	185	83.5	—	—
6/4	193.0	190	86.0	—	—

should always be kept cool (but never frozen), preferably in a domestic refrigerator.

WHAT ARE THE DIFFERENCES BETWEEN THE VARIOUS TYPES OF INSULIN?

Soluble (clear, regular) insulin consists of the pure hormone whose action has not been prolonged by any additive. Insulin used to be extracted only from beef pancreas. Nowadays, the main insulins used are either of pork origin, or synthesized artificially to exactly resemble human insulin. The length of action depends on the dose given but is rarely longer than 8-10 hours, so that three injections of this type of insulin would need to be given each day to adequately control the blood glucose level. The higher the dose, the greater and more prolonged the effect on blood glucose, and the same applies to all the other types of insulin described later.

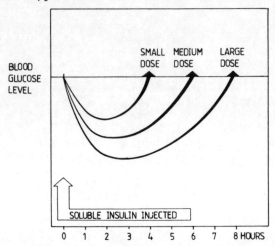

Insulin can be linked to various proteins which prolong its action to between 12 and 36 hours depending on the type and dose used. By contrast with clear, regular insulin, these **longer-acting insulins** are usually cloudy and mostly need to be given only once or twice a day. Some insulins are biphasic (mixture of short and long-acting insulins) and often provide better control.

SHORT-ACTING INSULINS

Insulin	Origin	Peak	Duration	Purity
		(Hours)		
Actrapid	Pork/human	3-4	6-10	Highly purified
Hypurin neutral	Beef	3-4	6-10	Purified
Velosulin	Pork/human	2-3	6-10	Highly purified
Humulin-S	Human	2-3	6-10	Highly purified

INTERMEDIATE-ACTING INSULINS

Insulin Name	Origin, mixed/biphasic	Peak	Duration	Purity
		(Hours)		
Semitard MC	Pork	6-8	14-16	Highly purified
Isophane	Beef	6-8	18-24	Standard
Hypurin Isophane	Beef	6-8	18-22	Purified
Insulatard/Hum	Pork/ Synthetic human	5-8	20-24	Highly Purified
Protaphane	Synthetic human	6-8	18-24	Highly purified
Lente	Beef/human	8-12	22-30	Standard/purified
Hypurin Lente	Beef	8-10	22-30	Purified
Lentard MC	Beef/pork	8-12	22-26	Highly purified
Monotard MC	Pork	8-12	20-24	Highly purified
Rapitard MC	Pork/beef	4-10	16-20	Highly purified
Mixtard/Human	Pork/ Synthetic human	4-6	20-24	Highly purified
Initard/Human	Pork/ Synthetic human	4-6	20-24	Highly purified
Humulin-I	Synthetic human	6-8	18-24	Highly purified
Human Monotard	Synthetic human	8-11	20-24	Highly purified
Actraphane	Synthetic human	8-12	20-24	Highly purified
Humulin M1-M4	Synthetic human	2-8	20-24	Highly purified

LONG-ACTING INSULINS

Insulin Name	Origin	Peak	Duration	Purity
		(Hours)		
Humulin ZN	Synthetic human	10-14	24-30	Highly purified
Hypurin Protamine Zinc	Beef	14-16	28-34	Purified
Human Ultratard	Synthetic human	10-18	28-34	Highly purified

Although different manufacturers produce very similar insulins, once control has been achieved, it is important to keep to the same manufacturer since minor differences may cause you to react differently. Always check the insulin carefully as soon as it has been dispensed by your pharmacy, since dispensing errors can occur.

Synthetic human insulins are being increasingly used, but probably carry no special benefits.

12/ AT WHAT TIMES SHOULD INSULIN BE GIVEN?

Insulin should always be injected 15-30 minutes before meals. The interval between the injection and the meal should be kept as constant as possible. Too early an injection may result in blood glucose levels falling too low before food is absorbed into the bloodstream: this is particularly important when short-acting insulins are being used. Too late an injection may result in blood glucose rising too high before the insulin has a chance to act. Both situations are clearly undesirable.

Once daily injections are rarely able to control the blood glucose level for a whole 24 hours. **Twice** daily injections (before breakfast and evening meal) often work well: a somewhat higher dose is usually needed for the morning injection. Mid-morning, mid-afternoon, and bedtime snacks are needed to "buffer" the action of insulin in both once and twice daily routines. Giving **three** short-acting doses each day, before meals, together with a medium or long-acting insulin at bedtime is proving to have big advantages: the doses can be changed from day to day to allow for different meal sizes and patterns of exercise. Timing of meals and exercise can also be much more flexible. Mid-morning and mid-afternoon snacks can be omitted (*although the bedtime snack is still essential*). Many people find that on this regimen, dose adjustments are easier to plan and more logical.

For some patients, insulin may be used in addition to tablets. Often, the way this is done is to take your sugar-lowering tablets through the day and have a single dose of one of the longer acting insulins either at night or in the morning. Your doctor will give you very individual advice if you are one of these patients.

 ## 13/ HOW DO I MANAGE SYRINGES AND INJECTIONS?

Syringes can be either glass or plastic disposable. Most people find the disposable plastic syringes preferable, and those with fixed needles are now almost standard.

Many doctors feel that a disposable syringe and needle can be re-used quite safely, but check with yours to be sure he agrees with this approach. If so, after injection, replace the syringe in its plastic envelope without rinsing it and keep it in the refrigerator. After five or six injections, a new syringe and needle should be used, although blunting of the needle may mean changing it more frequently.

Syringes vary both in capacity (½ or 1 ml) and in markings, which can be confusing. You should always confirm with your doctor or nurse exactly how the marks on the syringe correspond to the dose to be injected. The standard ½ ml syringe provides 1 unit for every mark: the 1 ml syringe provides 2 units for every mark.

A. Drawing up Insulin
1. Draw back the same amount of air into the syringe as the quantity of insulin you will need to draw up.
2. Inject air into the ampoule
3. Slowly, draw back the quantity of insulin required. If an air space or bubbles develop,

move plunger in and out until the correct amount of insulin, free of bubbles, is in the syringe. Then withdraw the needle. Different types of short and long-acting insulins are sometimes prescribed to be given at the same time. Draw up the clear insulin first, then the cloudy, and inject as soon as possible.

B. **Injection Technique** (which will be demonstrated by the doctor or nurse)

1. Cleaning the skin with spirit before injecting is no longer thought to be necessary. Spirit tends to toughen the skin, making injections more difficult and blunting your needles more quickly.

2. Injections should be given under the skin, not into it, using a needle no longer than ½" (1.2 cm). The injection should ideally be given at right angles (90°) to the skin surface, but certainly at no smaller angle than 45°. The needle can be inserted to the hilt.

3. With glass syringes, be sure that there is no leakage of insulin around the plunger while injecting.

4. Never use exactly the same spot twice in succession, although different spots no closer than 2-3 cm (1" apart) in the same area can be used successfully. Ideally, rotate the injection sites so that a different major area of the body is used for each injection. Repeated injections in the same area are more likely to produce swelling (hypertrophy) or occasionally loss (atrophy) of fat tissues at the site of the injection. However, the purity of the insulins which are now used makes this problem far less likely to occur.

5. Some stinging during the injections is usual; pain or burning after the injection, or irritation or reddening at the site of the injection are abnormal, and should lead to discussion with your doctor. The cause may be either faulty injection technique or an allergy to the type of insulin being used.

6. When going to your doctor or the pharmacy, always take both a syringe and an empty insulin package or ampoule along, to compare

this with what is being newly prescribed or supplied. This will help to avoid errors.

C. Placing of Injections
Every diabetic develops his or her personal routine, but the diagrams below show the range of possibilities.

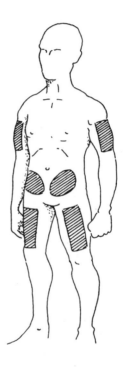

In some people, insulin seems to have a more rapid effect if injected into the arms than the legs, with a slower effect still from the wall of the abdomen. Your own experience may lead to the use of certain areas rather than others.

D. Insulin Pens
Many people now prefer to use pens which can be "loaded" with a cartridge containing 150 units of insulin. The dose can be "dialled-up" before injection, making for a simpler injection routine. The special needles are detachable, so that they can be changed as often as necessary. Most insulin types are now

available in cartridge form. It is a good idea to have a spare pen in reserve in case the one(s) you use are broken or mislaid. Over the next few years, pre-loaded pens will be increasingly used. Once empty, they are simply discarded, and a new one used.

14 / IS EXERCISE IMPORTANT?

Yes. Any form of exercise causes the muscles to use more glucose. Not only is the blood glucose level lowered immediately after exercise, but there appears to be a long term lowering of blood glucose in people whose lifestyle is more energetic. Taking exercise often means that you should reduce your insulin dose beforehand - or increase your intake of food. In some people, the blood-sugar lowering effect of insulin continues for many hours after the exercise. It may then be necessary to reduce the next dose of insulin to allow for this effect. Only trial and error will allow you to work out what is best for you.

Most people do not realise how inactive they really are. Tiredness and fatigue after a day's work are more likely to be due to emotional stress and tension than to the effects of muscular exercise.

Any type of exercise is satisfactory for diabetics, including cycling, regular sport, or just plain walking. A careful look at your lifestyle and discussion with friends and family should help you plan a more energetic way of life, whatever your age or other medical problems.

Remember that many factors can affect the

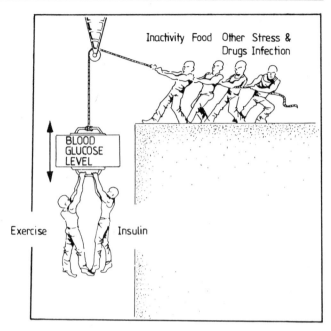

blood glucose level and the diagram above will remind you of the most important ones.

 ## CAN EXERCISE CAUSE ANY PROBLEMS?

Yes. If both food intake and insulin dose remain the same, a sudden increase in exercise can result in quite a sudden fall of blood glucose, producing an insulin reaction (hypoglycaemia or "hypo"). This is because exercising muscle uses up some of the glucose in the blood. In addition, if you exercise the legs (eg. cycling) after an injection into a leg, the insulin is absorbed into the circulation more quickly. This can lower the glucose level in the blood even further. The symptoms will be described later in this booklet (see Question 24). When exercising, hypos can be prevented by:

a) Eating a larger meal before, or nibbling during exercise

b) Reducing the insulin dose on immediately

21

preceding the planned exercise (e.g. game of squash) by an amount which your doctor will advise, or you will work out yourself by trial and error.

c) Always carrying lumps or cubes of sugar (or a glucose tablet such as Dextrosol) with you in case a "hypo" occurs, or to prevent one should the exercise prove longer and more severe than anticipated.

16/ WHAT IS THE "HONEYMOON" PHASE OF DIABETES?

In some diabetics, the insulin dose needed to control blood glucose falls during the first few weeks or months of treatment. Occasionally insulin needs to be stopped altogether. However, this is only temporary and does not indicate that your diabetes is cured. Watch your urine or blood tests carefully and be prepared to recommence the insulin. The cause of this interesting phenomenon is still not clear.

17/ WHY CONTROL DIABETES WELL?

It is not hard to put together a pattern of diet, insulin, and exercise in such a way as to avoid the symptoms of both hyperglycaemia (Question 3) and hypoglycaemia (Question 24) but this is not enough!

Particularly if you are young, with a long life span ahead, keeping blood glucose levels as close as possible to those of a non-diabetic has now been shown by many research workers to reduce the likelihood of getting the so-called complications of diabetes in later life. These are dealt with individually in Question 29.

Achieving good control requires a lot of your own involvement and thought, and your doctor will be glad to provide additional guidelines on the many small ways through which control can be improved.

18 / HOW CAN YOU TELL WHETHER YOUR DIABETES IS WELL CONTROLLED?

By the way you feel? No! This can be most unreliable. *Many diabetics may feel perfectly well despite having uncontrolled diabetes:* yet such a situation can produce undesirable effects over a period of time. However, the symptoms listed in Question 3 should be well recognised by you: if they occur, your diabetes is badly out of control! The cause must be found and corrected immediately.

By testing the urine? Yes! Every insulin-receiving diabetic should test their urine (or ideally their blood) once or more each day.

By testing the blood? Yes! Measuring the blood glucose is becoming more simple and is much more informative than testing urine. It can of course be accurately done in the laboratory. In addition, strips are available (such as Glucostix or BM 1-44) which, when covered by a drop of blood obtained by pricking your own finger or ear lobe, change colour according to the blood glucose level.

Small pocket-size and comparatively inexpensive meters are also available to measure blood glucose rather more accurately. These techniques enable you yourself to assess and control your own diabetes to a degree which was previously impossible. Your doctor or nurse will be happy to discuss these procedures with you.

Untreated or poorly controlled diabetes also raises the blood level of certain fats (lipids), including cholesterol and triglyceride. Your doctor may check the blood levels of these fats from time to time and may advise a change in diet if they are abnormal. There is considerable evidence to suggest that keeping blood fats at normal levels improves the long term health of arteries (see Question 29).

A blood test (called **haemoglobin A₁**) provides an estimate of average blood glucose over the previous two months or so, and helps your doctor to assess yet another aspect of control. More tests of this type are being gradually introduced into clinical use. A haemoglobin A_1 value above 8% usually means that there is room for improvement!

HOW ARE URINE AND BLOOD TESTED FOR GLUCOSE?

URINE TESTING: Clinistix (or **Testape**). These dip-strips are useful only for finding out whether glucose is present or not: they are not satisfactory for assessing the actual amount, and should not be used routinely by diabetics. **Diabur-5000** or **Diastix** dip-strips show a better and more definite colour change, depending on how much glucose is present. These are satisfactory for routine use. The results should be recorded as 0, 1/10, 1%, etc.

Ketodiastix, which enable you to measure ketone levels on the same "dip" are also available (see Question 26).

Whichever test you use, it is important that you very carefully follow the instructions which accompany the test kit: the length of the "dip" and the time at which you "read" the colour are both of the utmost importance.

Aspirin (in doses of more than 600 mg per day) or vitamin C (in doses of more than 250 mg per day) can affect the chemicals in the urine testing equipment. They can reduce the apparent sugar level when using strips and thereby make the urine test results look better than they really are.

BLOOD TESTING:

A small drop of blood, sufficient to produce a *proper* "blob" (not a smear) on the blood testing strip, is the first essential. Using a lancet in one of the readily-available "prickers" is the best way to get the blood painlessly and reliably. Use all the finger tips one-by-one to avoid soreness, and consider using the earlobes if fingers do get sore! Whichever the type of strip used, the *exact* moment that the blood comes in contact with the strip must be accurately noted (or the button on the meter pressed). When blood has to be wiped off the strip again, *accurate timing is essential.* If you use a meter, you can usually get "check fluids" to see if your meter gets the right reading. Or ask your doctor or nurse to check a blood sample in the laboratory from time to time to see if it matches your reading of the same blood sample. If you use a meter to read the sticks and get an unusually high (or low) reading, check the colour visually (if it is that sort of strip): the meter may be faulty!

20 / WHEN SHOULD TESTS BE DONE?

Urine tests: Before meals is the least likely time to show glucose; one to two hours after meals is usually the most likely time to show glucose. Your doctor will recommend one or both times and probably suggest a bedtime test as well on certain evenings. The object of urine testing is to obtain a clear picture of your control during waking hours, and 2 to 4 tests a day are usually necessary to provide this picture for you and your doctor.

Testing during the working day is useful, although possibly inconvenient. However, you can pass a sample into a small clean bottle (such as a well washed out tablet bottle), and test it when you get home later in the day.

The urine that you test has been produced

by the kidneys during the period since you last emptied your bladder; the early morning test therefore gives no information about control at that time, but only gives an idea of the average control through the previous night. To deal with this problem, "second sample" or "interval" testing is often recommended. In this procedure, urine is passed at say 7.00 am then again at 7.30 am, only the second sample being tested. This gives a better idea of the blood glucose at that particular time. The same procedure can obviously be used at other times of the day.

Blood tests: At least one blood test a day is advised; more often if you are unwell or when the diabetes is obviously not well controlled. Testing at different times each day provides a better overall picture for you and your doctor. If an unusual result is obtained, it is a good idea to check again at the same time for one or two further days: a dose adjustment may be needed.

Whatever method you use for testing, it is essential that you write down all your test results in a test record book and bring it to the clinic or doctor's surgery at each visit. In this way, your medical adviser can see exactly how you are getting on and can perhaps help you to improve your control. Without this information, your doctor or nurse can only give a fraction of the help that would otherwise be possible.

 ## WHAT IS A NORMAL BLOOD GLUCOSE LEVEL?

In people without diabetes, fasting blood glucose (after not eating overnight) is less than 5 millimoles per litre, or 90 milligrams per decilitre (shortened to mmol/l or mg/dl). After food, it rarely rises above 8 mmol/l (145 mg/dl). In untreated or uncontrolled diabetes, blood glucose may even rise above 30 mmol/l (540 mg/dl).

With treatment, your doctor will aim to keep your level at less than 10 mmol/l (180 mg/dl) for all or most of the time, and will in many cases help you to achieve the lower, more normal, levels mentioned above. It is important to emphasise that symptoms of hyperglycaemia (Question 3) rarely occur unless blood glucose is consistently higher than 14 mmol/l (250 mg/dl).

Therefore just because you feel well, it does not necessarily indicate that your diabetes is controlled.

 DO POSITIVE GLUCOSE TESTS IN THE URINE ALWAYS INDICATE POOR CONTROL? No! The amount of glucose which appears in the urine depends not only on blood glucose levels but also on the height of the kidney barrier to the "overflow" of glucose. It may help to compare this process to the function of a storage tank:

In non-diabetics, glucose rarely appears in the urine because this kidney barrier or "threshold" is normally 8-10 mmol/l (145-180 mg/dl: A in diagram) and as indicated earlier,

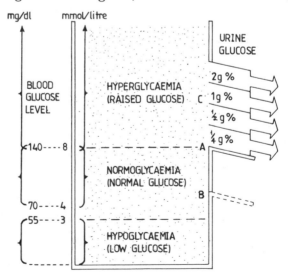

blood glucose of non-diabetic people does not usually exceed this figure.

The threshold is also normal (8-10 mmol/l) in many diabetics, so that absence of urine glucose *usually* means that the blood glucose is not above this level.

Some diabetics, however, have a low threshold for glucose (B in diagram), occasionally even as low as 4 mmol/l (70 mg/dl). This means that glucose overflows into the urine even with a normal blood glucose level. Should the urine be kept free of glucose all the time in this situation, you are almost certainly over-treating the diabetes, creating a real risk of producing hypoglycaemia. Pregnancy almost always produces a low threshold, so that urine tests become particularly unreliable as a means of assessing control in this situation.

On the other hand, some diabetics, particularly with increasing age or kidney disorder, have a high threshold (C in diagram). Blood glucose can then be quite high, without glucose appearing in the urine, giving a false impression of good control. It is for all these reasons that measurement of glucose in the blood is being recommended for most people.

23/ HOW CAN I ACHIEVE THE BEST POSSIBLE CONTROL OF MY DIABETES?

This challenge is probably one of the most important facing an insulin-dependent diabetic! It is not easy because our lifestyle varies so much during a single day, and from one day to the next. A normal pancreas adjusts to diet, exercise, and stress automatically, by changing its output of insulin. Being diabetic, *you* have to take over this function.

Firstly, always have three regular meals each day. A mid-morning and mid-afternoon snack are necessary if you are on a twice-daily insulin regimen. A before-bedtime snack is essential whatever insulin regimen has been advised for you. It won't hurt to go out for a meal which might be larger than usual, once in a while, but **anticipate** by taking more insulin beforehand. Being prepared to do finger-tip blood sugar tests after such an unusual meal will tell you whether you have adjusted your dose correctly. Remember that one hour after a meal, blood glucose should not exceed 10 mmol/l (180 mg/dl). The same **anticipation** applies to stress situations (examinations, performances, arguments, as well as infections of all types): don't wait for diabetes to go out of control, raise the dose first if you are able to anticipate the problem. Look again at the pulley diagram on page 21 to remind yourself of the factors which will affect your blood glucose level.

If you measure your blood glucose level often enough, you will learn to judge how much more insulin than usual you need for such situations.

The same **anticipation** is the keynote to handling exercise (see also Question 15). Drop your insulin dose by anything from 4 units to half of your usual dose before a game of tennis, a long hike, or a cycle ride. Taking some extra carbohydrate with exercise may of course suit you better. Always check your blood glucose level to see that you have done it correctly.

Remember that on two doses of insulin each day, your morning dose affects the blood glucose at midday and before the evening meal, while your evening dose affects the late night and early morning glucose levels. On four doses of insulin a day, each pre-meal dose affects the blood glucose about 4 hours later, and the bedtime dose affects the early morning blood glucose. Achieve before-meal blood glucose levels of 4-7 mmol/l (70-120 mg/dl) and after-meal levels of 7-10 mmol/l (120-180 mg/dl), and you can be very pleased with yourself.

Even if you get the most accurate blood glucose result, it will only improve your control if you act on it! Therefore do at least one or two tests a day, and record the results together with any unusual happenings (such as insulin reactions) in your test record book. Then, be prepared to adjust, as outlined above, all the variables of your lifestyle and insulin doses. If you get an unusual result, ask yourself at the time why you think it happened, and again write the reason down in your record book. It will help you to understand your diabetes better. Contact your doctor or nurse as often as you think necessary. Do not wait until your next appointment before getting this advice, otherwise you will have lost valuable time in terms of the health of your body.

WHAT IS HYPOGLYCAEMIA (INSULIN REACTION, OR "HYPO")?

When the blood glucose level falls below 3 mmol/l (55 mg/dl), the following symptoms may develop:

hunger	dizziness
sweating	faintness
palpitations	confusion and vagueness
trembling	loss of consciousness and fits
slurring of speech	

A "hypo" occurring at night may reveal itself only by restlessness, nightmares, and a headache the morning after. A positive ketone but negative glucose test in the first urine passed next morning is another clue to a "hypo" occurring during the previous night.

Every diabetic has a slightly different pattern of symptoms of hypoglycaemia: in fact your doctor may deliberately arrange to give you a "hypo" to help you recognise the symptoms, should they later occur.

After many years of having diabetes, the "early warning" hypo symptoms such as sweating, trembling and palpitations may be lost. The problem may also result from having your diabetes too well controlled! If this happens, you will need to be more alert to the other symptoms. A slight reduction of insulin doses or change of insulin type may be worth a try, after discussing it with your doctor: occasionally this maneouvre will restore the usual warning symptoms.

The main causes of hypoglycaemia are:
a) Late or missed meals
b) Accidental overdose of insulin
c) Increased physical activity, without an increase in food or a decrease in insulin
d) Drinking alcohol on an empty stomach.

Hypoglycaemia is therefore a preventable problem.

a) Late or missed meals should never occur, and the risks of hypoglycaemia are much reduced by ensuring that you have three proper meals together with a mid-morning, mid-afternoon and bedtime snack. (On a four-a-day injection routine, the meal snacks are not usually needed but the bedtime snack is still essential.)

b) Accidental overdose of insulin, if it does occur, can usually be dealt with by taking extra carbohydrate. However, if you realise that an accidental overdose has been given which exceeds the usual dose by more than half, contact your doctor immediately for advice.

c) Increased physical activity may not always be predictable, making it essential to have lump sugar, a Dextrosol tablet, or something similar at hand at all times (see Question 15).

d) When drinking alcohol (especially spirits), ensure that you eat at the same time.

The body has efficient built-in mechanisms for reversing mild to moderate hypoglycaemia, but these should never be relied upon to correct this abnormal situation. Repeated attacks of severe hypoglycaemia can result in brain damage. Therefore, frequent hypoglycaemia should immediately be mentioned to your doctor so that changes in insulin or diet can be carried out.

25 / HOW SHOULD HYPOGLYCAEMIA BE TREATED?

Firstly, **avoid hypoglycaemia** whenever possible. Always have lump (cube) sugar or Dextrosol in your pocket or handbag to correct minor hypoglycaemia should it occur. More severe hypoglycaemia should be promptly corrected by an immediate snack of sweetened milk and a biscuit (or cookie). Should you become drowsy and not able to take action yourself, your identification bracelet or pendant should enable others to provide force-feeding with a sweetened drink.

Failing this, a doctor will need to give you a glucose injection directly into a vein, and if no doctor is immediately on hand, no time should be wasted in having you transferred to the casualty department of the nearest hospital. From this point of view, your family, friends, employers, or other working colleagues should be made aware of the action they should take under such circumstances.

Glucagon, a hormone which has the opposite effect to insulin, is also available. If you tend to get severe episodes of hypoglycaemia, particularly if you live or are travelling remote from medical care, your doctor may supply ampoules of glucagon in a kit to be given to you in an emergency by a relative or friend. The usual dose is 1 mg (in 1 ml of solution) given in a syringe with a longer needle into the muscle of the upper arm, just below the shoulder. A feeling of sickness occurs in some people given glucagon.

WHAT ARE KETONES, AND HOW DOES ONE TEST FOR THEM?

Body fat is nothing more than an insulator and a reserve store of energy. If a person eats nothing for 12-18 hours, fat is broken down to provide this reserve energy. Some of the breakdown products of fat are substances called ketones, and these will appear in the urine under such circumstances, whether a person is a diabetic or not.

In the diabetic, however, ketones will also appear in the urine if diabetes goes badly out of control. This occurs because there is not enough insulin to provide the body cells with the energy (glucose) that they need: here again, the reserve energy (fat) stores are being called upon.

This is a serious warning!

Ketones are most easily tested by Ketostix strips or the combined Keto-diastix strips, so that glucose and ketones can be measured at the same time. Do the test whenever you feel ill in any way. If positive, do it again in four hours. If still positive, see your doctor **immediately**, or contact your "hotline" number.

WHAT ARE KETOACIDOSIS AND DIABETIC COMA?

If diabetic control remains poor, ketones cannot be excreted rapidly enough in the urine, and ketone levels will rise in the blood as well. Because ketones are acids, this affects the entire bodily function, and tiredness, drowsiness, sickness and vomiting can occur. In addition, by this time the large amount of glucose in the urine will cause an excessive loss of water. The mouth becomes dry, and breathing becomes deep and rapid. If no action is taken, coma develops.

This whole sequence rarely occurs in less than 24 hours, so that there is time to take avoiding action. Before the days of insulin, ketoacidosis was the major cause of death in diabetics. Today, provided ketoacidosis is identified and treated early, recovery is the rule. However, ketoacidosis is preventable.

Taking action!

If you are thirsty or passing more urine than usual, or show heavy (2%) urine glucose (or blood glucose over 17 mmol/l) at any time, you should immediately check for ketones. If positive, test the urine again in four hours. If still present, you must immediately contact your clinic, hospital or family doctor, unless you have been given other specific instructions on dealing with this situation (see Question 28 and 36 and 37).

 HOW CAN KETOACIDOSIS BE PREVENTED: SICK DAY RULES. There is always a good reason for the loss of control which leads to ketoacidosis:

Too much food or too little exericse

Too little insulin (forgotten, or incorrect dose)

Some medications such as cortisone-like drugs, water tablets (diuretics), etc.

Infection or other stress.

a) **Food and exercise problems:** These are easily prevented by either avoiding changes in eating and exercise patterns, or increasing the dose of insulin before problems arise. The amount by which you should increase the insulin is a matter of trial and error.

b) **Your insulin requirements** can change over a period of time. Showing consistently higher sugar should prompt you to increase the dose of insulin slightly (2-8 units) or, preferably, contact your doctor.

c) **A forgotten insulin dose** is not a disaster. If taking twice daily insulin, and you remember before your midday meal, give half to two- thirds of your usual dose then. If you only remember before your evening meal, check your urine or blood sugar and take advice on what dose you should give from either your doctor or your "hotline". If on four injections a day and you miss one of your doses, it will produce a rise of blood glucose which is unlikely to cause you a problem: it is not usually worth adjusting the other doses.

d) **Additional drugs** which you are prescribed should always be discussed with your physician to ensure that they do not interfere with diabetic control. Furthermore, some tablets (including aspirin and vitamin C) interfere with the chemical reactions in Diastix and other urine glucose test strips, although they do not actually affect the glucose content of blood or urine. Therefore, if you are taking any of these preparations regularly, you may get a mistaken idea of your diabetic control.

e) **Infection and stress** are unavoidable aspects of life. Any stress, whether physical (an accident), mental (worry or depression), or medical (operations, infections, or even a common cold), will cause some rise in blood glucose level to an extent which differs from person to person. In any of these situations, the insulin may need to be increased by anything from 2 units to double the usual dose as soon as (or preferably before) urine or blood glucose indicates a loss of control. You will get to know your own responses to these stresses, and discussion with your doctor will help to provide additional guidelines.

If your illness makes you vomit, feel sick, or you cannot eat, do not stop your insulin, keep giving the same dose: it may even need to be increased. Try to keep taking fluids which also provide some carbohydrate. The following foods may be useful if you are unwell because they provide concentrated carbohydrate in a liquid form to balance the effect of the insulin you are taking.

sugar	glucose
jam/honey/marmalade	Ribena (undiluted)
orange squash (undiluted)	orange juice
lemonade	Bournevita/ Ovaltine/
milk pudding (tinned)	drinking chocolate
Complan (powder)	Build-Up (powder)

If ketones appear, contact the "hotline" number immediately (see Question 36).

If you remain ill for as long as six hours, arrange for someone to take you to the closest hospital accident and emergency (casualty) department, at once.
If your diabetes is seriously out of control and you are away from medical care generally, you may need to use an emergency measure to keep yourself out of trouble, until medical advice is available. Give yourself 4 units of a fast-acting insulin such as Actrapid every hour, also checking your blood sugar hourly until your glucose level is normal. It is also important to keep your fluid intake high (about 1/2 to 1 pint of water per hour in the early stages).

WHAT ARE THE SO-CALLED COMPLICATIONS OF DIABETES?

Arteriosclerosis (hardening of the arteries) occurs to some extent in almost every person as they age, whether they are diabetic or not. In some diabetics, it may occur somewhat earlier than usual. Arteriosclerosis is the cause of stroke and heart attacks. It may also produce poor circulation in the legs which leads to painful calves on walking, ulcers on the feet, and occasionally gangrene.

Hardening of the arteries is caused by fat being deposited in the walls of the arteries, so that they become narrowed, and even blocked. From time to time, your doctor will check the level of cholesterol (as well as other fats) in your blood. Keeping these blood fat levels normal reduces the risk of developing heart attacks and strokes. The way to keep the fat levels normal is to keep to the recommended diet (see Questions 8 & 9). Somewhat stricter dieting and even medicines may be prescribed for you if the fats in the blood test are found to be above safe levels.

Diabetics should not smoke: smoking is the other big cause of hardening of the arteries. If arteries do become blocked, they can quite often be treated by a surgeon stretching or bypassing the block. But, prevention is better than cure!

Cataracts are degenerative changes in the lens of the eye which can cause dimness of vision. Cataracts occur commonly in non-diabetics and somewhat more frequently in diabetics, especially if blood sugar levels are allowed to run high. Cataract can be treated by quite a simple operation: the surgeon will usually replace your damaged lens with an artificial one.

Retinopathy is the name given to leaky and abnormally fragile small blood vessels in the retina, the seeing part of the eye. Such abnormalities may cause blurring, and occasionally loss of vision.

It is your responsibility to make sure that a doctor (or suitably qualified optician) checks over the retina of the eye every year with an ophthalmoscope. Even once retinopathy has developed, it can be treated by using laser beam therapy ... unless it is left too late!

Neuropathy signifies nerve damage, which can cause weakness, pins and needles, or a loss of feeling in the hands or feet, and occasionally dizziness and other unusual symptoms. Even impotence can occur in men, although this may be due to factors other than diabetes. If you have this problem, do mention it to your doctor: a number of treatments are available.

Nephropathy means kidney damage, which may occur after long-standing diabetes. It is for this reason that your doctor checks for protein in your urine when you visit him: if present, it may be an early sign of this problem. Some people may need dialysis (artificial kidney) treatment, or even a kidney transplant.

High blood pressure occurs rather more often in people with diabetes. It can help to cause heart attacks and strokes, and can also worsen retinopathy and nephropathy. You must make sure that your doctor or nurse checks your blood pressure at least once each year. Quite simple tablet treatment is available for this problem. If you are taking such tablets, make sure that your blood pressure is checked every three months or so. You should know what your blood pressure is, and also know what level your doctor is aiming for. It is generally accepted that a blood pressure above 160/90 is undesirable at any age: in some situations even lower targets are preferred.

Infection, particularly of the skin and urinary system, is more likely to occur in diabetics than in people without diabetes. In addition, healing of even minor injuries is sometimes slower.

All these complications can be effectively treated, particularly if detected early. It is for this reason that the doctor will make a systematic examination of various parts of your body approximately once each year. You may need to remind him that this annual review is due! Keeping your diabetes well controlled is also one way that you yourself can help minimise the risk of these complications.

DOES EVERY DIABETIC GET COMPLICATIONS AT SOME TIME?

No. There is good evidence that most of the above complications are less likely to occur if the diabetes is well controlled, and if weight gain is avoided. However, it must be admitted that even the best controlled diabetic sometimes does have one or other of the complications mentioned above, although usually in a milder form.

HOW IMPORTANT IS FOOT CARE?

A diabetic's feet can be very vulnerable. Nerve damage (neuropathy) can prevent feeling an injury, scratch, or cut; poor blood supply to the feet may then mean poor healing of the injury and infection or gangrene can develop.

The following rules are important to follow:

a) Avoid walking bare-foot, even at home

b) Do not cut your toenails too short, and cut nails to follow the line of the toe.

c) Never cut your own toenails if you have a

significant eye-sight problem, or a nerve or blood vessel disorder affecting the feet: see a state registered chiropodist regularly every 6-8 weeks, if possible.

d) Avoid tight shoes: preferably have new shoes fitted by an expert who knows you are diabetic.

e) Wash, dry, and examine your feet carefully at least every other day: even the most minor infection should be immediately discussed with your doctor.

f) Never attempt to treat any foot problem yourself. Permanent damage may result from the use of "over the counter" remedies: always seek professional advice first.

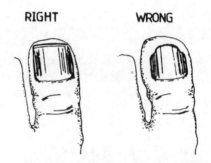

RIGHT   WRONG

If an ulcer, sore or other foot infection develops, do not delay: contact your doctor immediately.

32/ A FEW ADDITIONAL PROBLEMS

Can I smoke? Diabetes alone may damage the blood vessels of your body, as mentioned earlier. If you smoke as well, your chances of such damage are that much greater.

Can I drive a car? Yes, but the licensing authorities may want to have your doctor's reassurance that your diabetes is sufficiently stable, and that you are otherwise well: an appropriate form will need to be completed, on which you must mention that you have diabetes.

Can I play sport as usual? Yes (see Questions 14 and 15).

Can I drink alcohol? Yes, but as mentioned earlier, calories do count. In addition, if you are prone to having many "hypos", alcohol (especially spirits) may block the body's corrective responses, and make your "hypos" more severe. Remember that you should always have a carbohydrate snack if you have an alcoholic drink.

Does diabetes interfere with employment? Hardly. Jobs involving physical responsibility for other people (e.g. bus drivers, airline pilots, certain branches of the armed forces), or involving personal danger (working on high buildings, diving, etc.) are not suitable for insulin-receiving diabetics. Apart from these situations, there should be no problems. The earlier discrimination against diabetics is now almost non-existent since it has been shown that the work record of diabetics is on average better than non-diabetics.

Can I get life insurance? Yes. You may have to accept a "loading", but life assurance is possible for most diabetics. Shop around and seek the advice of your Diabetic Association office.

Can I have children? Yes. Diabetes is at least partly inherited. If either parent is a diabetic, the risk of any one child becoming diabetic at some time of their life is certainly greater than if this was not the case. However, the risk is not so high as to make having children unwise.

Pregnancy in a diabetic should always be managed by a physician/obstetrician team accustomed to dealing with diabetic pregnancies. If you are planning a family, let your doctor know. With your help, he will try to ensure that your control is as close as possible to perfection at the time you conceive: if you are practising contraception, he will advise you to continue until your control is just right. This is now considered to be important in reducing some of the problems which may occur in pregnancy.

Contraception: Most of the presently available low-dose pills are satisfactory for diabetics and there is no reason why you cannot use intra-uterine devices (IUD) or other contraceptive methods. If you are "on the pill", it is useful to stop it and to have one normal period before you conceive, so that the exact stage of pregnancy is known. Your physicians will be happy to discuss any other aspects of diabetes and pregnancy with you.

WHEN SHOULD I SEE MY DOCTOR OR CLINIC?

Routinely.......... Ideally you should have a discussion with him or her at least every 3-4 months. Do not forget to take your test record book with you when you go.

At about yearly intervals and perhaps more frequently, your doctor will systematically examine your eyes, blood pressure, heart, blood vessels on the feet, and check for nerve damage. He will not mind if you remind him that your 12 months check is due. He or she will test the urine for protein and check the level of control of your diabetes and your kidney function. He may also take blood to see whether the blood fat (cholesterol and triglyceride) levels are normal. An alteration to the diet, and perhaps tablets, may be suggested if they are not. As indicated earlier, a number of drugs in everyday use for other conditions may affect the control of your diabetes, or interfere with the strip tests. Therefore, at these visits ask your doctor for reassurance that none of the other drugs that you are taking are interfering in any way. Each time you see either your family doctor or specialist, it is useful to take along your syringe or pen injector (it may need checking), your diet sheet (it may need changing), and your urine or blood test record book (so that the doctor has information on the basis of which he may recommend any change in treatment).

In an emergency............ If your tests show high sugar levels consistently, or if you begin to feel thirsty or unwell, do not wait: get advice. Make sure that you have one or more telephone numbers that you or your family or friends may contact for advice on such unexpected problems, and write them down in the space provided on page 44 (Question 36 "Hotline").

 IDENTIFICATION Always carry a card, or better still, a bracelet or pendant, indicating that you are a diabetic. In this day and age, accidents will happen, and it is obviously important that anyone can immediately identify you as being diabetic. The Medicalert Foundation (local address available from your doctor), which provides identification bracelets and pendants at a modest cost, now has branches in many countries. This system is highly recommended. Alternatively, have your local jeweller make up one for you.

 FINALLY Remember that knowing about your diabetes is your responsibility. Your doctor, dietitian, clinic sister, or chiropodist/podiatrist will be only too happy to answer queries and suggest further reading material.

Membership of the British Diabetic Association has much to offer. It can help you follow recent trends in diabetes care. Much research is also being carried out in diabetes, including new methods of giving insulin, and in transplanting the insulin-producing parts of the pancreas. You will find it useful and interesting to keep in touch with these and other important developments. If you are a youngster or teenager, the Association provides group activities in which you may enjoy participating.

36 / "HOTLINE"

In this space a telephone number should be written, from which you can get advice 24 hours a day, seven days a week, should any sudden problem occur which affects your diabetes. Your doctor will advise you which number to insert.

....

37 / OTHER IMPORTANT CONTACT NUMBERS

Your family doctor ....

Your clinic appointment clerk ....

Your dietitian ....

Your chiropodist/podiatrist ....

Your diabetic advisory service ....

/38/ SOME BOOKS FOR FURTHER READING

Insulin Dependent Handbook.... by John Day.
Publishers: Medikos
Diabetes at your Fingertips...... by Peter Sonksen,
Charles Fox and Sue Judd. Publishers: Class
Publishing
Diabetes - a Basic Guide.... by Rowan Hillson.
Publishers: McDonald Optima